Mediterranean Diet for Beginners

A diet plan, for meals prep, with 7
practical recipes throughout the week
To lose weight, live healthy and fit

GILLIAN WILLET

Table of Contents

Introduction

The Mediterranean diet is the name that has been given to a particular dietary regimen that was originally used by people in poorer regions of Italy and Greece for many centuries. This diet was not originally thought to be particularly healthy in these regions, as the people ate these foods because of necessity, rather than because of the Mediterranean diet weight loss and excellent nutrition benefits they experienced. This type of cuisine is far different from what you might expect from this region, but it is overall much healthier because things like lard and butter are rarely used.

In recent years, a growing number of men and women in different countries around the world have become increasingly concerned about their health. Because of the fact that many people have become more concerned about their overall health, these men and women have paid closer attention to what they eat on a regular basis. In the final analysis, these men and women are making dietary decisions designed to improve their general health and wellbeing.

As people have become more conscious of their health and diet, a considerable number of these same men and women have become interested in the Mediterranean diet regimen. If you are, in fact, a person who appreciates the interrelationship between diet and health, you may have a definite interest in the history of the Mediterranean diet regimen.

Before you can appropriately understand what the Mediterranean diet is all about, you need to appreciate that it is more of a concept than a specific dining routine. In reality, there is no such thing as a Mediterranean diet common to all of the countries in the Mediterranean region of the world. Rather, the "Mediterranean diet" consists of those food items that people who live in the various nations in the region consume in common.

Chapter One

History Of The Mediterranean Diet

The Mediterranean Diet is steeped in the culinary traditions of the Mediterranean region, particularly Greece and Italy. The importation of the diet into America and other parts of the world began in the 1940s and '50s.

The Mediterranean tradition offers a cousine rich in colors, aromas and memories, which support the taste and the spirit of those who live in harmony with nature. Everyone is talking about the Mediterranean diet, but few are those who do it properly, thus generating a lot of confusion in the reader.

And so for some it coincides with the pizza, others identified it with the noodles with meat sauce, in a mixture of pseudo historical traditions and folklore that do not help to solve the question that is at the basis of any diet: combine and balance the food so as to satisfy the qualitative and quantitative needs of an individual and in a sense, preserves his health through the use of substances that help the body to perform normal vital functions.

The purpose of our work is to demonstrate that the combination of taste and health is a goal that can be absolutely carried out by everybody, despite those who believe that only a generous caloric intake can guarantee the goodness of a dish and the satisfaction of the consumers. That should not be an absolute novelty, since the sound traditions of the Mediterranean cuisine we have used for some time in a wide variety of tasty gastronomic choices, from inviting colors and strong scents and absolutely in line with health.

The Mediterranean diet has its origins in a portion of land considered unique in its kind, the Mediterranean basin, which historians call "the cradle of society," because within its geographical borders the whole history of the ancient world took place.

The origins of the "Mediterranean Diet" are lost in time because they sink into the eating habits of the Middle Ages, in which the ancient Roman tradition - on the model of the Greek - identified in bread, wine and oil products a symbol of rural culture and agricultural (and symbols elected of the new faith), supplemented by sheep cheese, vegetables (leeks, mallow, lettuce, chicory, mushrooms), little meat and a strong preference for fish and seafood (of which ancient Rome was very gluttonous).

The rich classes loved the fresh fish (who ate it mostly fried in olive oil or grilled) and seafood, especially oysters, eaten raw or fried. Slaves of Rome, however, was destined to eat poor food consisting of bread and half a pound of olives and olive oil a month, with some salted fish, and rarely a little meat.

The Origins of the Mediterranean Diet

The concept of the Mediterranean diet is derived from the eating habits and patterns of the people who populate the countries of Italy, Greece, Spain, France, Tunisia, Lebanon and Morocco. As a result, the Mediterranean diet actually includes a tremendous array of delectable food. In point of fact, if a person elects to adopt the concept of the Mediterranean dining scheme, or if a person elects to follow a Mediterranean diet regimen, he or she will have the ability to enjoy a remarkable assortment of scrumptious fare.

The diet of the peoples that have populated the regions around the Mediterranean Sea actually have remained nearly completely unchanged for well over one thousand years. The history of the region is replete with examples of men and women living longer than similarly situated people who consumed alternate diets. Through the centuries, the people of the Mediterranean Sea region have enjoyed longer lives that people in other parts of the world at the same historical epoch.

At the heart of the Mediterranean diet are foods and beverages that are indigenous to the geographic landmass surrounding the Mediterranean Sea. In short, the development of the Mediterranean dieting and dining pattern initially developed by providence. The people of the region naturally and understandably ate those foods and drank those beverages that readily were available in and around their homes.

The Historical Elements of the Mediterranean Diet Scheme

As mentioned previously, over the centuries, the diet of the peoples of the Mediterranean Sea region has remained essentially unchanged. The Mediterranean diet consists of the bountiful consumption of a number of healthy food items including:

* Fresh fruit

* Fresh vegetables

* Low fat nuts

* Whole grains

* Monounsaturated fat

In a similar vein, the Mediterranean diet utilized by people for generation after generation excludes or limits certain food items that have been deemed harmful in recent scientific studies. These less than desirable food items include:

* Saturated fats

* Red and fatty meat

* Rich dairy products

* Fatty fish

Chapter Two

The Mediterranean Diet

By its name alone, the Mediterranean diet attracts a lot of current and would be dieters due to its exotic name. But what is it exactly? One concern of the Mediterranean diet is that it allows 40% fat consumption. Let's go into more detail as it seems a waste to just let it go without giving it a fair reading.

The Mediterranean diet evolved from the respective diets of countries surrounding the Mediterranean basin. Among the countries surrounding the basin are the south of France, southern Italy, Spain, Portugal, Greece and Cyprus. Based on scientific data, people around the Mediterranean basin had lower rates of cardiovascular disease compared to Americans who, for all intents and purposes, consumed the same relative amount of fat.

One possible explanation is the presence of olive oil and red wine. Olive oil lowers cholesterol levels in the blood, while red wine contains flavonoids. Flavonoids are anti-oxidants that also help the body when dealing with allergenic material, viruses and cancer causing agents.

Another contributing factor to a European's better health could be the fact that they tend to walk more than Americans do. Questions have also been raised as to whether the Mediterranean diet contributes enough iron and calcium to the diet. Green vegetables and goat cheese have been found to contribute these nutrients respectively.

The thing about the Mediterranean diet is that its foods are often rich and tasty thanks to olive oil. Normally, margarine and hydrogenated oils lack the flavor that olive oil gives out. Another part of the diet is regular but moderate consumption of red wine. Saturated fat consumption is low as opposed to high amounts of monounsaturated fat and dietary fiber. This is due to the fact that the diet includes big servings of fruits, vegetables, breads, cereals, olive oil and fish.

Characteristically speaking, the Mediterranean diet has high consumption of olive oil. Breads, cereals, fruits and vegetables likewise have a high rate of consumption in the diet. Fish and poultry as well as wine are moderately consumed, while eggs and red meat are rated as very low in consumption.

The problem with most diets is that they tend to be extreme. Some diets, like the vegetarian diet, limit a person to just eating fruits, tofu, yogurt and vegetables. Other diets would require high protein intake while severely limiting intake of the other food groups. Like a user friendly computer, the Mediterranean diet does not go to extremes to achieve a desired result. The diet allows for consumption of tasty foods. This allows the dieter to actually enjoy the gastronomic delights normally prohibited by other diets. A solid testament to this fact rests on the presence of wine in the diet.

The most surprising aspect of the Mediterranean diet is that fat is regarded as a healthy dietary component. Keep in mind that it is the fat that gives food most of its flavor. Two substances, omega-3 fatty acids and monounsaturated fats, are considered to be healthy and are not restricted in the diet. Olive oil, canola oil and nuts are good sources of monounsaturated fat while fish, vegetables and nuts contain the healthy omega-3 acids.

Saturated fats and trans-fat, on the other hand are considered to be unhealthy as they contribute to heart disease. Red meat, butter cheese and milk are sources of saturated fat while processed foods contain hydrogenated oils from which trans-fat comes from.

The Mediterranean diet emphasizes: Eating primarily plant-based foods, such as fruits and vegetables, whole grains, legumes and nuts. Replacing butter with healthy fats such as olive oil and canola oil and using herbs and spices instead of salt to flavor foods.

FAST FACTS ABOUT THE MEDITERRANEAN DIET

There is no one Mediterranean diet. It consists of foods from a number of countries and regions including Spain, Greece, and Italy.

The Mediterranean diet is a great way to replace the saturated fats in the average American diet.

There is an emphasis on fruits, vegetables, lean meats, and natural sources.

It is linked to good heart health, protection against diseases such as stroke, and prevention of diabetes.

Moderation is still advised, as the diet has a high fat content.

The Mediterranean diet should be paired with an active lifestyle for the best results.

The Mediterranean diet is a way to ensure food comes from a range of natural, healthful sources.

The Mediterranean diet consists of:

- High quantities of vegetables, such as tomatoes, kale, broccoli, spinach, carrots, cucumbers, and onions
- Fresh fruit such as apples, bananas, figs, dates, grapes, and melons.
- High consumption of legumes, beans, nuts, and seeds, such as almonds, walnuts, sunflower seeds, and cashews
- Whole grains such as whole wheat, oats, barley, buckwheat, corn, and brown rice

- Olive oil as the main source of dietary fat, alongside olives, avocados, and avocado oil
- Cheese and yogurt as the main dairy foods, including Greek yogurt
- Moderate amounts of fish and poultry, such as chicken, duck, turkey, salmon, sardines, and oysters
- Eggs, including chicken, quail, and duck eggs
- Limited amounts red meats and sweets
- Around one glass per day of wine, with water as the main beverage of choice and no carbonated and sweetened drinks

This focus on plant foods and natural sources means that the Mediterranean diet contains nutrients such as:

Healthful fats: The Mediterranean diet is known to be low in saturated fat and high in monounsaturated fat. Dietary guidelines for the United States recommend that saturated fat should make up no more than 10 percent of calorie intake.

Fiber:

The diet is high in fiber, which promotes healthy digestion and is believed to reduce the risk of bowel cancer and cardiovascular disease.

High vitamin and mineral content:

Fruits and vegetables provide vital vitamins and minerals, which regulate bodily processes. In addition, the presence of lean meats provides vitamins such as B-12 that are not found in plant foods.

Low sugar:

The diet is high in natural rather than added sugar, for example, in fresh fruits. Added sugar increases calories without nutritional benefit, is linked to diabetes and high blood pressure, and occurs in many of the processed foods absent from the Mediterranean diet.

It is difficult to give exact nutritional information on the Mediterranean diet, since there is no single Mediterranean diet. This is because a variety of cultures and regions is involved.

Benefits

The Mediterranean diet is not specifically a weight loss diet, but cutting out red meats, animal fats, and processed food may lead to weight loss.

In areas where the diet is consumed, there are lower rates of mortality and heart disease, and other benefits.

Diabetes

The Mediterranean diet can help protect people from type 2 diabetes and improve glycemic control.

Several studies have shown that those who follow a Mediterranean diet have lower fasting glucose levels that those do not.

Basically, a Mediterranean diet calls for people to eat a great deal of fresh fruit, plant foods, fish, poultry, some dairy products, while using extra virgin olive oil as the primary source of fat. Also, a moderate amount of eggs can be eaten each month, while red meat is to be avoided as much as possible. Red meat can be eaten in low amounts, but meals should not be centered around it because of how it affects the heart.

The Mediterranean diet is meant to lower the risk of heart disease, since olive oil is high in monounsaturated fats, which have been known to reduce this risk substantially. This also reduces the body's cholesterol levels, which is also a positive thing for the body.

THE CONCEPT OF THE MEDITARRANEAN FOOD PYRAMID

For most of us, the most recognized symbol of healthy food is found in the food pyramid. It indicates which foods we should eat in which portion sizes so that our body receives the nutrients it requires. If you're creating a healthy diet plan you would do well to look at the Mediterranean diet food pyramid. The Mediterranean diet is recognized as one of the healthiest diets in the world and is actually endorsed by the Mayo Clinic.

What is the Mediterranean Diet Food Pyramid?

The Mediterranean diet food pyramid is an alternative to the traditional one which is becoming increasingly popular because it is not based on popular food trends. The diet itself is founded on thousands of years of tradition within the Mediterranean region. The dietary traditions of Mediterranean countries have long been recognized as very healthy, and the food that they consume is one of the main factors in that healthiness. Knowing the difference between the traditional food pyramid and the Mediterranean one will assist you in improving your health.

The Mediterranean diet food pyramid is significantly different to the traditional one with which we are familiar. There are certain glaring differences, namely;

- The Mediterranean one does not have a fats category
- Red meat is at the top of the Mediterranean pyramid as a food to

eat least of all along with sweets/desserts.

- Olive oil is grouped with the fruits and vegetables as something to be consumed frequently

The top portion of the Mediterranean diet food pyramid starts with red meat as a source of animal protein. Red meat and sweets are the least consumed foods in the Mediterranean, around 2-3 times per month. The next category, consumed a couple of times per week, are poultry, eggs and dairy products like cheese and yogurt. Next comes fish and seafood which are consumed almost daily. Basically, the Mediterranean diet is low in saturated fats and high in monounsaturated fats and omega 3.

The bottom level of the pyramid is composed of fruits, vegetables, legumes (beans), nuts, seeds, herbs, spices, whole grain bread, whole grain pasta, couscous, brown rice, polenta and other whole grains. People in the Mediterranean rarely eat processed grains (i.e. white flour). A large variety of these fresh foods are eaten daily, and they are usually either raw or lightly cooked. This means that the nutrients are still intact. Cooking foods actually kills most nutrients or renders them undigestible. Hence, it is always better to eat food raw or partially cooked.

The final part of the Mediterranean pyramid is the recommendation of six glasses of water per day and a moderate amount of wine (i.e. one glass of red wine with dinner).

It is interesting to note that olive oil is grouped with the fruit and vegetables in the Mediterranean pyramid. As you can imagine, olive oil is a large part of the Mediterranean diet and many dishes contain it. While it is true that oil is high in calories, olive oil is a healthy monounsaturated fat which is high in antioxidants and contains omega 3 so we can consume a little more as long as we don't go overboard.

Monounsaturated oils like olive oil are anti-inflammatory and are good for diseases like asthma and arthritis. They're also heart healthy because the omega 3 lowers LDL ("bad") cholesterol, and raises HDL ("good") cholesterol. The most healthy olive oil is extra virgin olive oil.

You may be wondering how people in the Mediterranean receive their iron since they don't eat a lot of red meat. The answer to this is the same as it would be for a vegetarian. Legumes (beans) and green leafy vegetables are also good sources of iron and the Mediterranean diet is full of these healthy foods. In fact, the whole Mediterranean diet food pyramid consists of healthy foods ensuring that those who follow the Mediterranean diet experience optimum health.

Mediterranean Food Pyramid

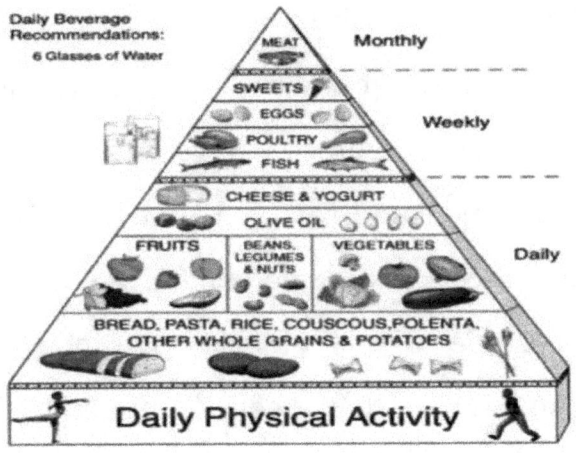

The main concepts of the Food Pyramid are the "proportionality", that is the right amount of foods to choose from for each group, the "portion" standard quantity of food in grams, which is assumed as the unit of measurement to be a balanced feeding, the "variety", i.e., the importance of changing the choices within a food group, and "moderation" in the consumption of certain foods, such as fat or sweets.

As you can see, at the base of the pyramid are grains, followed by fruits and vegetables, legumes, olive oil, low-fat cheese and yogurt, which should be eaten daily. Meat is not excluded, but is given the preference to that of chicken, rabbit and turkey rather than beef. Along with fish and eggs should be eaten only a few times a week, for the supply of high quality protein. Beef or red meat should be eaten only a few times a month.

Each group includes foods, which are substantially "equivalent" on the nutritional plan, in the sense that they provide nearly the same type of nutrients. It is obvious that, within the same group, foods despite being homogeneous with each other can have small differences in terms of quality and quantity of patrimony in nutrients.

However, this does not affect the concept of "interchangeability" of foods. The latter in fact, if they belong to the same group, being nutritionally equivalent, may be substitutes for each other, without, however, affecting the adequacy of the diet, provided you comply with the variety. In nature does not exist a "complete" food, i.e. it contains all the nutrients the body needs, and that is why it is necessary to vary as much as possible food choices and properly combine foods from the different groups.

A very varied diet not only avoids the risk of nutritional imbalances and possible consequent metabolic imbalances, but it also satisfies the taste of fighting the monotony of flavors. Each group expected is represented by at least a portion of the foods that constitute it, to vary the choices within the same group.

Understanding The Mediterranean Diet

The Mediterranean Diet is not a diet per se but a loose term referring to the dietary practices of the people in the Mediterranean region. Each country that borders the Mediterranean Sea offers a variant to the Mediterranean Diet. Differences in ethnic background, culture, agricultural production, and religion between the Mediterranean countries creates the variation in each country's diet. However, each diet offers a number of characteristics that are common to all of the Mediterranean countries.

The Mediterranean Diet has a high consumption of fruits, vegetables, beans, nuts, seeds, bread, and other cereals. Traditionally, fruits and vegetables are locally grown in the Mediterranean Diet. Fruits and vegetables often are consumed raw or minimally processed. Fruits and vegetables contain many essential vitamins and minerals as well as antioxidants that are crucial for good health.

The Mediterranean Diet's primary source of fat is in the form of a monounsaturated fat. Olive oil is a monounsaturated fat that is a rich source of antioxidants including vitamin E. Olive oil is used instead of butter, margarine, and other fats. In fact, butter and cream are only used on special occasions. Olive oil in the Mediterranean

Diet is used to prepare tomato sauces, vegetable dishes, salads, and to fry fish.

The Mediterranean Diet encourages moderate intake of fish but little to no intake of meat. Red meat and poultry are consumed only sparingly. Fish is the meat of choice. About 5-15 oz. of oily fish, in particular are consumed weekly. Oily fish includes tuna, mackerel, salmon, trout, herring, and sardines. Oily fish are a great source of omega-3 fatty acids.

Dairy products are consumed in low to moderate amounts. Dairy products from a variety of animals such as goats, sheep, buffalo, cows, and camels are primarily consumed in the form of low fat cheese and yogurt. Very little fresh milk is consumed.

Meals are usually accompanied by wine or water.

The Mediterranean Diet encourages low to moderate consumption of wine. Wine is usually consumed with a meal. The type of wine consumed is usually red wine which contains a rich source of phytonutrients. Among the phytonutrients, polyphenols especially are powerful antioxidants. Studies have shown that men and women who have a light to moderate consumption of alcohol live longer than nondrinkers. One alcoholic drink (1.5 oz. distilled spirits, 5 oz. wine, 12 oz. beer) daily for women and two alcoholic drinks daily for men is considered moderate intake of alcohol.

If you are looking to incorporate the Mediterranean Diet into your life, here are a few suggestions. Fruits and vegetables should be of a wide variety. You should try for at least 7-10 servings of whole fruits and vegetables daily. You should avoid any vegetables that are prepared in butter or cream sauces. High fiber breads, cereals, and pasta are consumed daily. This includes brown rice, bran, whole grain bread and cereal. You should avoid sweets, white bread, biscuits, breadsticks, and any refined carbohydrates.

Protein intake is low in saturated fat. Protein intake from red meat is of lean cuts, poultry without the skin, and low fat dairy foods (skim milk, yogurt). You should avoid bacon, sausage, and other processed or high fat meat. You should also avoid milk or cheese that is not low fat.

Intake of fish is 1-2 times weekly from oily fish, flaxseed, walnuts, and spinach. Healthy oils (extra virgin olive oil, canola oil, flaxseed oil) are used for cooking, salad dressings, and other uses. You should avoid omega-6 oils such as corn, sunflower, safflower, soybean, and peanut. Your diet should also include peas, beans, soybeans, lentils, tree nuts (almonds, pecans, walnuts, Brazil nuts), and legumes. You should avoid heavily salted or honey roasted nuts.

A moderate intake of alcohol with the evening meal is optional. The Mediterranean Diet emphasizes whole natural foods. This means avoiding fast food, fried food, margarine, chips, crackers, baked goods, doughnuts, or any processed foods that contain trans fatty acids.

The Mediterranean style diets are very close to the dietary guidelines of the American Heart Association. Diets of the Mediterranean people contain a relatively high percentage of fat calories, about 40%. The American Heart Association endorses a diet that contains about 30% fat intake. However, the average Mediterranean Diet has less saturated fat than the average American diet.

Researchers are now trying to deduce the components of the Mediterranean Diet that are responsible for the Mediterranean populations' longer life expectancy compared to other European populations. However, the combined effects of different ingredients such as a relaxed eating attitude, plenty of sunshine, and more physical activity are likely to be contributing to the overall healthy lifestyle of the Mediterranean region. The Mediterranean Diet has a lower incidence of heart disease and cancer, which makes the Mediterranean Diet an overall good choice in health.

FOCUS OF THE MEDITERRANEAN DIET

The main focus of the Mediterranean Diet is actually on vegetables, fruit, unrefined carbohydrates such as root vegetables and wholegrain cereals (refined carbohydrates being things like bread, cakes, pasta and refined cereals). It is also high in fibre, and low in sugar and saturated fat. This describes the Mediterranean Diet in a nutshell. Once you successfully incorporate this in your routine, you certainly won't go wrong. Part of it is their approach to meat. The focus is less on red meat and more on poultry and seafood.

In general, people in the Mediterranean only eat red meat a few times per month but they eat poultry at least once per week and fish and seafood even more often. As you can imagine, this reduces their cholesterol levels significantly because of the Omega 3 in the fish, hence the reduction in heart disease risk. They also eat dairy products daily like goat's cheese and yogurt.

Quite obviously, lower cholesterol levels are the first step toward heart health. But where do we get cholesterol from? Cholesterol comes from saturated (bad) fats found in dairy foods and meats. Another contributing factor to heart disease is sodium (salt), although our body needs sodium, in western society we tend to consume too much sodium. As much as possible, avoid foods high in the saturated fats found in meat and dairy, when eating red meat, try to have lower fat options.

What is the Mediterranean diet's answer to this? The secret is food high in healthy polyunsaturated and monounsaturated fats like those found in seafood, and olive oil. These also contain plenty of Omega 3 fatty acids which actively reduce cholesterol levels. Omega 3 fatty acids are found in fatty fish. Popular varieties in the Mediterranean diet include sardines, whitebait, salmon, tuna, herring and mackerel. Other popular Mediterranean seafood choices include mussels, crab, shrimp, red mullet, squid, swordfish and sea bass.

There are many health benefits to following a Mediterranean diet. The people of the Mediterranean have a much lower incidence of cancer, heart disease, stroke, diabetes and even things like Alzheimer's as a result of their diet compared to those of us in western societies. All of these things lead to to living a long and healthy life.

The final secret of the Mediterranean diet is a healthy exercise regime. While most acknowledge the importance of exercise, very few people actually maintain a regular exercise routine. It doesn't have to be anything strenuous, a 20-30 minute walk per day is sufficient. But many of us are too lazy to do this, we'd rather rely on the car. Or we feel that we are too busy to find time to exercise. But think of it this way, if we don't find time, we'll LIVE less time!

Chapter Three

Why The Mediterranean Diet Is A Healthy Choice In The 21st Century- Nutritionist And Doctors Review

₁f you are a person who has been on the hunt for a solid diet plan, you may feel overwhelmed much of the time. In the 21st century it is nearly impossible for a person to turn on a television set or open a newspaper without being bombarded with advertisements for a variety of different diet plans and products.

With the tremendous array of diet plans, programs, supplements and aids on the market, it can seem nearly impossible to select a diet plan that can and will best meet your needs now and into the future. More importantly, it can be hard to discern if one or another of these various diet schemes actually is a healthy course to pursue. In many instances, fad diets really are not based on the fundamentals of healthy living.

As you go forward considering what type of diet plan or regimen will best serve your interests and improve your health into the future, you will want to take a look at the benefits that can be had through the Mediterranean diet.

While there are multiple reasons why the Mediterranean diet is a healthy approach, there are five primary reasons why the Mediterranean diet is a good choice.

1. The Benefits of Fruits, Vegetable, Fiber and Whole Grains

A major component of the Mediterranean diet includes the regular consumption of fresh fruits and vegetables. Medical experts and nutritionists universally agree that a person should eat between five and six servings of fresh fruits and vegetables (or steamed items) on a daily basis.

People who adhere to the Mediterranean diet actually end up eating more than the minimum recommended allowance of fruits and vegetables. As a result, nutritionists in different parts of the world have taken to recommending a Mediterranean based diet regimen to their clients. Similarly, doctors who consult with their patients about healthy eating practices oftentimes find themselves recommending the Mediterranean diet in this day and age.

Beyond fruits and vegetables, the Mediterranean diet includes healthy amounts of dietary fiber and whole grains. Fiber and whole grains have proven effective in lowering the incidence of heart disease and some types of cancer.

2. The Benefits of Olive Oil -- Avoiding Saturated Fat

Some people have a fundamental misperception about the Mediterranean diet. These people have heard that the Mediterranean diet is high in fat. On some level, there is some truth in the conception that the Mediterranean diet is higher in fat than are some other dieting programs. A person following the Mediterranean diet does take in about thirty percent of his or her daily calories from fat. (Most diets recommended the intake of calories from fat at the rate of about thirteen to fifteen percent per day. However, these diets are contemplating the ingesting of animal fat.)

The vast majority of fat that a person on the Mediterranean diet consumes comes from olive oil. In other words, the fat found in the Mediterranean diet is not the dangerous saturated fat that can cause disease, obesity and other health concerns. In fact, research has demonstrated that there are a number of solid benefits to consuming olive oil, including a reduction of the risk of the incidence of breast cancer in women.

3. Dairy in Moderation

While the consumption of low or non-fat dairy products in moderation can be beneficial in some instances, many people the world over rely on heavy creams, eggs and other fat filled dairy products in their daily diets. The Mediterranean diet is low in dairy. Indeed, any dairy products that actually are included within the diet regimen is low fat. A person is considered an extremely heavy egg eater if he or she consumes four eggs in a week.

4. Red Meat in Moderation

Very little red meat is included within the Mediterranean diet. When it comes to meat items, this diet relies on moderate amounts of lean poultry and fresh fish. As a result, people who follow the Mediterranean diet plan have lower levels of "bad" cholesterol and higher levels of "good" cholesterol.

In addition, because of the inclusion of lean, fresh fish in the diet, adherents to the Mediterranean diet enjoy the anti-oxidant benefits that are found in certain fish oils and products.

5. A Well Balanced Dieting Scheme

In the final analysis, the Mediterranean diet is gaining acclaim from experts and adherents the world over because it is a balanced dieting program. Study after study demonstrate that a balanced diet that is low in fat and that includes fruits, vegetable, whole grains and lean meat works to ensure total health and wellness.

In recent years, doctors, researchers, scientists and nutritionists have taken a close look at the Mediterranean diet. Nearly universally, these experts and professionals have come away from their examination of the Mediterranean diet with positive perceptions of the dieting scheme.

There are a number of reasons why experts of all sorts -- from doctors to researchers to nutritionists -- look favorable upon the Mediterranean diet regimen. By considering the benefits of the Mediterranean diet that have been identified by experts, you will be able to better determine if the Mediterranean diet is right for you.

1. Low in Saturated Fat

On the surface, a person giving only a cursory review of the Mediterranean diet might conclude that it is not a healthy diet plan because it is "high in fat." Concluding that the Mediterranean diet is high if fat and harmful is an erroneous conclusion.

While it is true that the Mediterranean diet does derive a significant percentage of its calories from fat (around thirty percent daily in most instances), the calories come primarily from olive oil and consist of unsaturated fats. In other words, being low in saturated fat, doctors are recommending the Mediterranean diet for their patients.

2. A Plentiful Array of Fresh Fruits and Vegetables

Doctors are recommending that their patients eat at least six servings of fruits and vegetables throughout the course of the day. Many of these same doctors are turning to the Mediterranean diet because as a matter of routine people who follow this diet program are eating more than the minimum recommended daily allowance of fruits and vegetables. Additionally, rather than using processed fruits and vegetables, the Mediterranean diet features an abundance of fresh fruits and vegetables.

3. Low in Red Meat

Many doctors can be found encouraging their patients to limit the amount of red meat that they include in their diets. Limiting red meat in a diet can assist in lowering the levels of "bad cholesterol," helping to reduce the indigence of heart disease and some cancers.

4. Low in Fatty Dairy Products

Another reason that doctors favor the Mediterranean diet is found in the fact that the diet plan is low in the consumption of fatty dairy products. More and more doctors are encouraging their patients to use only low fat or non fat dairy products. People who follow the Mediterranean diet actually use very little dairy on a day to day basis. For example, a heavy egg eater on the Mediterranean diet eats four eggs a week. Many do not eat eggs at all.

In addition, milk is used within the diet in limited fashion. Heavy creams and sauces are not on the Mediterranean menu at all.

5. Helpful in Preventing Diseases

One of the primary reasons that doctors recommend the Mediterranean diet for their patients rests in the fact that the diet program has been demonstrated as being helpful in reducing the risks of certain diseases, including:

- Cancer
- Heart disease
- Cardiovascular disease
- Hypertension
- Diabetes
- Obesity

6. A Ready Source of Fiber and Whole Grain

Finally, doctors recommend the Mediterranean diet for their patients because it is high in dietary fiber and whole grains. Both fiber and whole grains have proven important in preventing disease and in maintaining an overall sense of wellness and good health.

The main ingredient in a Mediterranean diet that is believed to have the most influence on a person's health is extra virgin olive oil. This is because the diet is inherently low in saturated fat, but the olive oil makes it high in monounsaturated fat, which (as previously mentioned) is good for your heart. The Mediterranean diet is also very high in dietary fiber, which promotes regularity of the digestive system. The diet can sometimes be high in salt, when is contains:

- Olives

- Capers
- Salad dressing
- Fish roe

This salt content is not necessarily a negative thing, however, because those items contain natural salts the body can use and absorb more comfortably.

Exercise

One thing that many people might not realize about Mediterranean diet weight loss is that the people who originated the diet generally worked outdoors and reaonably hard. This means they were getting plenty of exercise each and every day, in addition to fresh air. This, in combination with the small portions these individuals would eat, led to very lean and muscular bodies. This assisted heart health of course, which is another reason why they suffered far fewer deaths from cardiovascular problems.

Medical Findings

A number of medical studies have been conducted on the Mediterranean diet and they have found that men who lived in Crete, which is one of the regions where this diet was originally used, had a low incidence of heart disease. This occurred despite the fact they actually consumed high amounts of fats in many cases. One of the main reasons for this finding is that many of these men switched from butter to extra virgin olive oil because it was less expensive. They also had a high vitamin C intake and reduced the amount of red meat compared to other parts of the globe.

It should be noted that the findings of this study were so dramatic that the results were published before the study had been completed. This was because the people who were conducting the study did not believe they could keep the information to themselves any longer. Other diseases and illnesses which have been positively affected from this diet include osteoporosis, minimising the risk of some forms of cancer, allergies, alzheimers disease and there are more studies being undertaken.

Weight Loss

Further studies have shown instances of Mediterranean diet weight loss, as 322 people participated in an experiment where some people were subject to a low-carb diet, others undertook a low-fat diet, and some ate only a Mediterranean diet. The results showed that those who were on the Mediterranean diet had the greatest weight loss of all, with the top two participants losing 12 and 10 pounds respectively. The study highlighted that Mediterranean diet weight loss is effective and should be considered by anyone who is having trouble losing weight.

Chapter Four

Mediterranean Diet Health Benefits

The Mediterranean diet has many health benefits. Wondering researchers have spent years trying to discover why. Although many regions have adopted a much more westernized diet habit which has resulted in a mounting obesity issue, communities that still follow the traditional Mediterranean diet continue to experience health which is the envy of the western world.

The Mediterranean diet consists primarily of fresh, healthy plant food like whole grains, vegetables, fruits, nuts, legumes, olives, fish and seafood. They combine this with reduced amounts of red meat and dairy products.

The Mediterranean diet is more nutritious because foods are less processed. Processing food, and even cooking it, deprives it of nutrients. But in a traditional Mediterranean diet, most foods are eaten raw or lightly cooked. When red meat is served it is usually trimmed of excess fat. The overall diet provides plentiful fiber, healthy fats, vitamins, minerals, protein and essential fatty acids required by the body to maintain health and prevent chronic illnesses like heart disease and cancer.

Another notable aspect of the traditional Mediterranean diet is that not every meal contains animal flesh (i.e. meat or fish). There are commonly days with no animal flesh being consumed at all. On these days, the protein portion of the meal is derived from things like beans, nuts, seeds and eggs. Although eggs are still animal products, recent research indicates that eggs do NOT increase blood cholesterol as scientists and doctors used to believe. Another modern day alternative to meat is tofu which comes from soy beans. While this is not a part of the diet, it would certainly be a worthwhile addition to it.

All of these things result in the Mediterranean diet being high in monounsaturated fatty acids, otherwise known as M.U.F.As which are healthy fats. Diets containing M.U.F.As (and polyunsaturated fats, or P.U.F.As) rather than saturated and trans fats, tend to provide certain health benefits including reduced risk of:

- Heart disease
- High Cholesterol
- Stroke
- Cancer
- Type II Diabetes
- Parkinson's Disease
- Alzheimer's
- Depression
- Metabolic syndrome

Lets take a closer look at these.

Reduced risk of heart disease and high Cholesterol

High levels of saturated fats result in increased cholesterol in the bloodstream. Over time, the cholesterol attaches to the walls of arteries causing a narrowing of the arteries that can lead to blockages, heart attacks and heart disease. Quite clearly, the reduced amount of saturated fat in traditional Mediterranean diets results in lower cholesterol levels. In some cases, high cholesterol is hereditary and is caused by the liver producing too much. A healthy diet containing high amounts of Omega 3 fatty acids is proven to actively combat this issue and can have a significant lowering effect on cholesterol levels.

Reduced risk of Diabetes

Consumption of complex carbohydrates and high fiber foods reduces the Glycemic Index of foods and low GI foods prevent spikes in blood sugar levels. So a low GI diet such as the Mediterranean diet tends to prevent diabetes. See the section on Metabolic syndrome below.

Reduced risk of Parkinson's & Alzheimer's

Some studies indicate that people who adhere to the Mediterranean diet have lower rates of Parkinson's and Alzheimer's diseases. Researchers are unsure why this is the case, but they believe that healthy food choices improving cholesterol, blood sugar levels and blood vessel health may be the cause.

Reduced risk of Depression

British Researchers studied depression and diet in more than 3,000 middle-aged office workers for five years. Their findings indicated that people who ate a diet high in processed meat, chocolate, sugar, fried food, refined cereals and high-fat dairy products were more likely to suffer depression. But people who ate a diet rich in fruits, vegetables and fish similar to a Mediterranean diet were less likely to suffer depression. Their findings support other research that has found that healthy diets can protect against disease.

Reduced risk of Metabolic syndrome

Many overweight and obese people suffer from a condition called Metabolic Syndrome. Metabolic syndrome is a group of conditions - high blood pressure, a abnormal blood sugar levels, excessive body fat around the waist or abnormal cholesterol levels - that occur together. These increase the risk of heart disease, stroke and diabetes. People on the Mediterranean diet have been found to be less likely to be overweight, thus reducing incidence of this condition.

A study showed that 13 thousand and 380 people who followed the Mediterranean diet, had a lower 83 per cent risk of diabetes type II, compared with those who did not bother using that system seriously. The research found that eating according to the Mediterranean diet leads to an improvement in cases of joint pain, and reduce the risk of pulmonary embolism, as well as reduce the risk of recurrence of colon cancer.

We do not know all the mechanisms that make a healthy Mediterranean diet completely, but research assumes the existence of a number of factors. And one reason only, the monounsaturated fat in olive oil and fish, have anti-inflammatory effects, which may help in the prevention of heart disease, and many other diseases.

The fiber in whole grains and legumes can help for digestion, and maintaining disciplined levels of blood sugar. The fiber also creates a feeling of fullness, a sense reduces the appetite - and this is one of the levers to reduce the increase in weight. The other elements in a vegetarian diet also have influences on the cellular level, and the aging process, the process of development of cancer, and the process of the body's response to chemotherapy.

Well, of course, eating according to the Mediterranean diet excludes many of the foods that are known to cause health problems such as saturated fat from animal sources, trans-fat and refined carbohydrates.

The Mediterranean diet has several advantages. The elements are already available, and can be prepared easily and quickly, the food varied and delicious taste. And dealt with after meals, it will not let you feel hungry or deprived. Use plenty of vegetables that almost are rich in nutrients and low in fat and calories. It is rich in fiber, and saturated with elements of health-promoting.

The key here is diversity; you must deal with different kinds. Instead of exposing them to steam or boil, try grilled or placed in the oven. Make salad a main dish for you, with the addition of nuts and small pieces of chicken or fish, and grated cheese. Eat plenty of fruits, vegetables, such as it is, a few in the caloric value of general and saturated nutrients, and antioxidants, and fiber.

Most fruits naturally have sweet taste, so it can serve as a snack or a great substitute for sweets and a meal. Type of fruit; definitely put them over the power. At breakfast in the morning you can eat whole grains or products with milk, yogurt and berries or pieces of banana. Eating nuts which contain a lot of antioxidants and other nutrients, For example, nuts contains «Omega-3» fatty acids, which reduce the risk of heart disease and blood vessels, and has adverse effects on the aging of the brain and skin.

Unlike the light products made from refined grains or mixed with refined sugar, the nuts have a function pointer a little sugar. However, the nuts are high in calories, so they fill up the hunger. Therefore, try not to deal with more than a handful of them (160 to 180 calories) per day. Sprinkle cooked vegetables from the veggie list with almonds. Dip fish or chicken with olive oil and crushed nuts, before grilling. Eat whole grains, which contain mostly carbohydrates that we need for energy consumption.

However, refined grains, such as white pasta, white rice, white bread, chips and products such as cornflakes and refined snacks, are virtually devoid of nutrients, including fiber cereal flakes. With little or no fiber therein, which slows digestion, the refined grain causes sudden increases in the blood sugar level.

Over time, this may lead to weight gain, heart disease and other disorders. Whole grains are rich in vitamins, minerals and proteins and have an influential role in the stability of the level of blood sugar. Perhaps you are now addressing bread from whole grains, brown rice, oats, but there are plenty of other delicious options.

Chapter Five

Mediterranean Diet & You

The Mediterranean diet is best for your heart. It is the way to eat and drink to your health. It is rich in vegetables, grains (rice, pasta), fish, fruit and dried beans.The Mediterranean diet is a wonderfully healthy diet and an extremely easy one to adapt to our stressful and fast paced lifestyles.

This diet is a balanced diet full of a variety of foods and can be followed easily. A main factor in the appeal is its rich, full flavored foods.It is also very low in saturated fat and includes plentiful amounts of fresh fruits and vegetables.

Another reason why the Mediterranean diet is good for you lies in the fact that the diet includes the consumption of a significant amount of fruit and vegetables.

Whether you want to lose weight, lower your cholesterol, eat more fruits and vegetables, or just feel healthier in general, adopting a Mediterranean diet is a great way to eat better while enjoying a delicious variety of food.

The Mediterranean diet is low in red meat and hence the diet plan works to reduce the amount of bad cholesterol.

The Mediterranean diet is high in whole grains and fiber as well as in anti-oxidants. It is also low in dairy products.

LONGEVITY

The history of the people of the Mediterranean region demonstrates that the Mediterranean diet works to extend a person's life.

The Mediterranean diet is one of the most suggested nutritional behaviors of the world. Adherence to it is associated with a significant reduction in mortality.Recent news reports that the Mediterranean diet is preferable for people suffering from diabetes over a low-carb diabetic diet.

There are a number of reasons why it is proving itself to be good for men of all ages.

In addition to assisting men in fighting obesity and bringing their weight down to a healthy level, the Mediterranean diet is effective in aiding men to maintain a healthy weight over time.

In fact, the Mediterranean diet is simply closer to what people have eaten for millennia.

Numerous studies have shown that the low-fat, high-fiber Mediterranean diet is one of the best recipes against health problems such as arthritis, obesity, diabetes, asthma and cardiovascular disease.

In fact, the latest research now shows that Spain is at the top of the European longevity league tables and it is widely believed that the Mediterranean diet is responsible for this.The main oil used in the Mediterranean diet is olive, traditionally cold pressed virgin, and this is used not only for cooking and in salads, but also for putting on bread in place of butter.

Olive oil

Olive oil rather than butter or cream is the primary source of fat in Mediterranean diet. Olive oil is often used alone or in substitution for other oils, butter, and margarine.

It is rich in a type of fat that readily converts to a fatty acid similar to omega-3. Olive oil is used as the primary cooking oil in Italy and Greece, and is a source of monounsaturated fat, which is much easier for the body to break down.

Olive oil, produced from the olive trees prominent throughout Portugal, Greece, Croatia, Turkey, Italy, Spain and other Mediterranean nations, adds to the distinctive taste of the food.

Olive oil also offers several health advantages over more polyunsaturated vegetable oils. Olive oil compounds also increase enzymes that block activation of carcinogens and improve their removal from the body.

Olive oil is also a good source of antioxidants. It contains anti oxidant Oleic acid that reduces the risk of breast cancer. It also contains vitamins A, B1, B2, C, D, and K, and Iron Poli-phenols.

Olive oil has been associated with lower blood pressure, a lower risk for heart disease, and possible benefits for people with type 2 diabetes.

Foods are cooked with extra virgin olive oil and enjoyed with small amounts of red wine. Instead of cooking with butter and spreading it on foods, use olive oil or canola oil.

But unlike the saturated fats that we commonly eat (such as butter, margarine, vegetable oil, trans fats) the primary fats of the Mediterranean Diet consist of monounsaturated fats (found in Olive Oil) which provide the health benefits for your heart.

The research shows that wine is better than beer or spirits at protecting against heart disease, that olive oil can reduce the risk of bowel cancer and that garlic may lower cholesterol levels.

Vegetables

The Mediterranean diet is one that is rich in vegetables, grains (rice, pasta), fish, fruit and dried beans. The other important factor is to make the consumption of fruits and vegetables a daily habit.

The vitamins, minerals, photochemical and fiber provided by the diets large amounts of vegetables, fruits, grains and beans are believed to account for the inhabitants of the Mediterranean countries lower incidence of cancer otherwise commonly found in the United States.

The Mediterranean diet emphasizes intake of fruits and vegetables, whole grains, nuts, and legumes.

Substitute a changing array of fresh vegetables and legumes for rice and potato side dishes.

Fruits

Typical fruits consumed in Med diet are: apples, pears, oranges, Mandarin, apricots, peaches, grape, water-melons, melons, raspberries, strawberries, chestnuts, walnuts, nuts, almonds, and pistachio nuts.

People who follow the Mediterranean diet and consume generous servings of fruits and vegetables each day have a lower incidence of certain diseases, including cancer and cardiovascular ailments.

Nuts

Nuts, legumes, and beans are consumed daily.

Most of the studies have focused on the Mediterranean diet, emphasizing the consumption of high amounts of virgin / extra virgin olive oil (up to one liter per week) or nuts (up to 30 grams a day, or two handfuls), in comparison to a low-fat diet.

Foods like vegetables, nuts and monosaturated fatty acids are very beneficial for the heart.

But if you eat a reasonable amount of calories and swap out candy bars for nuts, the data says you will be healthier.

The Mediterranean diet shifts towards more plant-based nutrition, as well as proteins from sources like beans and nuts rather than red meats.

Some of the desirable food items:

Bread, pasta, rice,

Vegetables: Spinach, Cauliflowers, Carrots, Eggplants, Tomatoes, broccoli, capsicum, capers, garlic and onion

Fruit: Olives, Grape, Oranges, Lemons, Apples, cherries, Strawberries, peaches, apricots

Legumes: beans, peas

Nuts: Walnuts, Almonds, Pistachio nuts

Oil: olive

Honey

Milk and cheeses

White Meat (chicken, rabbit, turkey, etc...) and

Fish (fish sword, sardines, tuna, clears)

Eggs

Red meat (veal, lamb, etc...) (consume less)

Walnuts contain polyphenols and other anti-oxidants and essential fatty acids. Abundant vegetables, fiber-rich beans, fresh breads and healthy fats found in olives and nuts are the mainstay of this region and essential to everyone's good health and vitality.

The Mediterranean Diet is now recognized as one of the healthiest diets in the world.

REASONS WHY THE MEDITERRANEAN DIET IS GOOD FOR YOU

Low in Saturated Fat

Physicians and nutritionists the world over all agree that a diet that is high in saturated fat can have very negative consequences on a person's health and wellbeing. Indeed, a diet that is high in saturated fat can cause a person to suffer heart disease, can lead to cancer and can cause a whole host of other health problems and concern.

The Mediterranean diet is noteworthy because of the fact that it is very low in saturated fat. The typical person who follows the Mediterranean diet intakes less than eight percent of his or her calories from potentially harmful saturated fat. This is significantly below the average of people who do not follow a Mediterranean diet regimen.

Includes Plentiful Amounts of Fresh Fruits and Vegetables

Another reason why the Mediterranean diet is good for you lies in the fact that the diet includes the consumption of a significant amount of fruit and vegetables. Indeed, the diet encompasses more fresh fruits and vegetables than any other dietary program or plan today.

Fresh fruits and vegetables have a significant beneficial effect on a person's health and wellbeing. People who following the Mediterranean diet and consume generous servings of fruits and vegetables each day have a lower incidence of certain diseases including cancer and cardiovascular ailments.

High in Whole Grains and Fiber

A benefit in the Mediterranean diet is found in the fact that it lowers in the incidence of certain types of cancer. One of the reasons that the Mediterranean diet lowers the incidence of cancer is found in the fact that the diet is rich in whole grains and dietary fiber. Both whole grain and fiber have proven to lower the incidence of cancer, including colorectal cancer.

High in Anti-Oxidants

The Mediterranean diet is high in anti-oxidants. Anti-oxidants play a significant role in maintaining the body -- including organs, muscles and skin -- in top condition. A diet high in anti-oxidants is believed to ensure that a person will live a longer, healthier life.

Low in Red Meat

Because the Mediterranean diet is low in red meat, the diet plan works to reduce the amount of "bad cholesterol." A diet low in "bad cholesterol" lessens the incidence of cardiovascular disease, hypertension and stroke.

High in Lean Meats

The Mediterranean diet includes lean meats in moderate portions. The reasonable amount of lean meats -- including fish and certain seafood and fish -- provides a health source of protein and energy for a person.

Low in Dairy

The Mediterranean diet is low in dairy products. In fact, a true adherent to the Mediterranean diet includes almost no dairy products at all. Any dairy that is included in the diet is low fat or non-fat. Because the diet is low in dairy, particularly fatty dairy products, the diet encourages a person to obtain or maintain an ideal weight. Additionally, the diet aids in reducing cholesterol and works to prevent heart disease.

Prevents Disease

As mentioned, one of the reasons that the Mediterranean diet is good for you rests in the fact that the diet plan appears to reduce the incidence of certain diseases including:

- Heart and cardiovascular disease
- Cancer
- Diabetes
- Hypertension
- Diabetes

Longevity

The history of the people of the Mediterranean region demonstrates that the Mediterranean diet works to extend a person's life. In addition, while working to extend a person's life, this diet scheme works to ensure that a person's longer life will be healthy as well.

3 IMPORTANT EFFECTS OF THE MEDITERRANEAN DIET

Significant research studies have been undertaken since 1970 designed to isolate the benefits of the Mediterranean diet scheme. While the research into the possible benefits of the Mediterranean diet is ongoing and not yet complete, scientists, researchers and nutritionists from around the globe have concluded from their extensive research that the Mediterranean diet is beneficial on a number of levels:

1. Reducing the incidence of certain diseases
2. Increasing longevity
3. Providing for an overall healthier lifestyle

The Mediterranean Diet and Disease Risk Reduction

Over the course of the past thirty years, a significant amount of research has been undertaken to consider the possibility that the Mediterranean diet might be useful in lowering the incidence of certain types of diseases. A number of significant studies have been undertaken in this regard, including research that has included an analysis of the dining habits in people in different countries around the world over time.

These studies initially were motivated by the fact that the people who populate the region surrounding the Mediterranean Sea tended to have lower incidents of different types of serious diseases that are on the increase in many different countries around the world. In this regard, researchers wanted to determine whether the reason the people of the Mediterranean region seemed to enjoy better health was environmentally driven or the result of their particular diet regimens.

These studies have demonstrated that Mediterranean diet appears to be effective in lowering the incidence of certain types of diseases:

1. Cancer (including breast cancer and colorectal cancer)
2. Coronary Disease
3. Other Cardiovascular Disease
4. Hypertension

The Mediterranean Diet and Increased Longevity

Of course, it goes without saying that if a person is able to reduce the risks of certain diseases through his or her diet, that person has a far better chance of living a longer life. In addition, it has been demonstrated that the substantial benefits of the Mediterranean diet have a cumulative effect on and for the human body.

What this means is that the longer a person follows the dining practices of the peoples of the Mediterranean region, the more ingrained the benefits of the diet become within the body. In simple terms, by utilizing and practicing the Mediterranean diet over time, a person will enjoy lasting benefits that will prolong his or her life.

By way of example, one might consider the negative consequences of smoking. If you elect to smoke cigarettes over a long period of time, you will cause irreparable harm to your body. Conversely, if you diligently follow the guidelines of the Mediterranean diet over time, your body will enjoy definitive and lasting benefits that will include good health and a longer life.

The Mediterranean Diet and Your General Health

Research has demonstrated that people who follow the Mediterranean diet are afflicted with fewer minor ailments such as colds and the flu than are their counterparts who follow other types of dining routines. In short, and on many levels, research over the course of three decades that people who follow a Mediterranean diet are afflicted with fewer illnesses, have more energy and suffer from the effects of being overweight or obese far less often than people who utilized other dietary practices.

WHY THE MEDITERRANEAN DIET IS GOOD FOR WOMEN

Over the course of the past forty years, women the world over have become particularly concerned about their diets. They have become concerned about diet related issues for two primary reasons:

1. Women have expressed concern over how a particular diet plan effects their appearances

2. Women have expressed concern over how a particular dies plan effects their health

As a result, a growing number of women have found themselves attracted to the Mediterranean diet. When it comes to the Mediterranean diet, there are six primary reasons why women find themselves strongly attracted to the diet regimen.

3. Weight Loss and Healthy Weight Maintenance

In many countries around the world, a record number of women are being classified as overweight and even obese. As a result, a growing number of women find themselves seeking effective and healthy dieting regimens to lower their weight to appropriate levels -- for both cosmetic as well as health reasons.

The Mediterranean diet has proven itself to be very effective at providing a means through which women can lose weight in a healthy manner. Additionally, the Mediterranean diet has proven incredibly effective as being a solid path a woman can take to maintain a generally ideal and healthy weight.

4. Anti-oxidants and Aging

The Mediterranean diet regimen is flush with foods that are rich in anti-oxidants. This includes leafy, dark green vegetables as well as certain fish that are common features in this dietary scheme.

Anti-oxidants have been proven to slow the appearance of aging in women. Additionally, anti-oxidants have been demonstrated as being effective at preventing organ and skin deterioration in women. The consumption of foods that are high in anti-oxidants has been proven to enhance longevity in both women and men.

5.Metabolic Syndrome

Metabolic syndrome is an ailment in which a person ends up afflicted with both Type Two diabetes and hypertension. Most experts believe that diet can play a significant role in reducing the likelihood of metabolic syndrome in men and women who are prone to the ailment.

Without exception, medical experts who have studied the cause and effect of metabolic syndrome universally have agreed that the Mediterranean diet is the perfect dietary scheme to prevent and control metabolic syndrome.

6. Heart Disease

Multiple studies in a number of different countries have concluded that the adoption of the Mediterranean diet lowers the incidence of heart disease in women (and men). Indeed, an analysis of the incidence of heart disease in the Mediterranean nations suggests that the use of the Mediterranean diet can lower the incidence of heart disease in women from twenty-five to forty percent.

7. Hypertension

Recent scientific studies have examined the rising incidence of hypertension amongst women. Many researchers attribute the increase in hypertension amongst women in recent years to a number of changes that have occurred in their lives, including:

- A greater number of women entering the workforce
- A growing number of women being forced to juggle the raising of children with a full-time career

- The food and beverage choices that women are making in the 21st century

Research studies in a dozen different countries over the course of the past twenty years have suggested that the Mediterranean diet is effective at lowering the incidence of hypertension in men and women. Because the Mediterranean diet is high if fruit, vegetables and whole grains and because the diet is low in saturated fats, most nutritionists and other experts believe that the dietary scheme works to lower hypertension in both men and women.

The Mediterranean diet combined with regular exercise has been demonstrated to have a marked effect on reducing the incidence of hypertension amongst middle-aged women.

8. Breast Cancer

Perhaps the most important "ingredient" of the Mediterranean diet is olive oil. Save for fresh fruits and vegetables (in most instances) olive oil universally is present in the Mediterranean diet. As a result, on the surface, the diet scheme appears to be high in fat. Indeed, upwards to thirty percent of the caloric intake of the Mediterranean diet does come fat. What is important to keep in mind is that nearly 100% of the fat in the Mediterranean diet is unsaturated and comes directly from olive oil. In other words, the fat in the Mediterranean diet essentially is healthy. Olive oil, and the fat contained in the product, simply does not trigger the negative consequences that flow from saturated fats, from animal fats.

In addition, there have been several important scientific studies undertaken in the past decade that have demonstrated that a diet high in olive oil works to lower the risk of breast cancer in women. Thus, one of the beneficial results of adopting the Mediterranean diet is a lowering of the risk for breast cancer.

THE MEDITERRANEAN DIET IS GOOD FOR MEN

One of the primary concerns of a growing number of men the world over is finding a diet and exercise plan that will assist in ensuring that they are in optimal health. In recent years, a significant number of men have found themselves attracted to the Mediterranean diet. These men have come to learn that the Mediterranean is a solid choice for assisting them in developing a comprehensive regimen for health living.

There are a number of reasons why the Mediterranean diet is proving itself to be good for men of all ages.

1. The Mediterranean Diet Reduces the Risks of Some Serious Diseases

Over the course of the past thirty years, a number of research studies have been conducted pertaining to the Mediterranean diet regimen. These studies have produced results that demonstrate that the Mediterranean diet can prove effective in reducing the incidence of a number of serious diseases and ailments in men.

The diseases in men that the Mediterranean diet appears to help prevent include:

- Cancer
- Heart and cardiovascular disease
- Hypertension
- Gallstones
- Stroke
- Diabetes

2. The Mediterranean Diet is Effective in Helping Men Reach and Keep an Ideal Weight

Many men are confronting problems related with being overweight and obesity. Indeed, in some countries, obesity is becoming the number one health concern amongst men of all ages.

Because the Mediterranean diet includes the consumption of generous portions of fresh fruits and vegetables, whole grains and lean meats, the diet can be very effective in assisting a man in bringing his weight down to a healthy, ideal level.

In addition to assisting men in fighting obesity and bringing their weight down to a healthy level, the Mediterranean diet is effective in aiding men to maintain a healthy weight over time. While it is one thing for a person to be able to lose weight, it is a completely different challenge for a man to be able to keep weight off over the long term. The Mediterranean diet has proven itself time and again as being a solid dietary program through which a person can maintain a healthy weight.

3. The Mediterranean Diet -- Adding Years to a Man's Life

Throughout history, the males who have populated the region in and around the Mediterranean Sea have been found to live lives longer than their counterparts in other parts of the world. In time, experts in the field of nutrition were able to demonstrate that men in the Mediterranean region lived longer because of their diets.

Scientists and other researchers have been able to demonstrate that there are positive, cumulative effects associated with the Mediterranean diet. In other words, by utilizing and following the Mediterranean diet over time, a man's life (in many instances) will be extended. In addition to having the chance to live a longer life because of dietary decisions, a man's life will be healthier and more robust because of his adherence to the Mediterranean diet scheme.

Chapter Six

Longevity And The Mediterranean Diet

Over the course of many generations, observers have been able to discern that the people who populate the region around the Mediterranean Sea live longer lives than do men and women in some other parts of the world. Historically, the reason most often attributed to the longevity of the people of the Mediterranean region was climate.

However, as researchers became more adept and as scientific methods became more sophisticated, it became clear that while the weather patterns of the Mediterranean area generally were pleasant and inviting, it was the diet of the people in the region that accounted for their longer lives.

There are a number of specific factors related to the Mediterranean diet that nutritionists and medical experts believe contribute to longevity. The more important of these elements are discussed within the confines of this article for your information and guidance.

1. Restorative Effects of the Mediterranean Diet

Many of the specific food items that are part of a Mediterranean diet regimen are high in anti-oxidants. Scientifically speaking, anti-oxidants are important compounds found in certain foods and beverages that work to neutralize the destructive nature of oxidants or free radicals that are found in the human body. Oxidants or free radicals are produced when the body burns oxygen to produce energy. In other words, oxidants really can be considered waste that pollutes the human body.

Over time, the accumulation of oxidants in the body accelerates the aging process. Cells wear and lose their elasticity. Organs end up functioning less efficiently and effectively. Indeed, recent scientific research has demonstrated that oxidants clog arteries raising the threat of stroke. Oxidants are found to contribute to cancer, heart disease and diabetes -- the major diseases most responsible for causing people to have premature deaths.

The types of fruits and vegetables that form the foundation of the Mediterranean diet -- including richly colored and leafy green vegetables -- which are high in anti-oxidants, have a restorative and life prolonging effect on the typical human body.

2. Reducing Cancer Risks

In most parts of the world, cancer of various types is the leading cause of premature death. Studies undertaken by researchers in Europe, Japan and the

United States in the past thirty years have demonstrated that the Mediterranean diet effectively reduces the risks of certain types of cancers.

A diet that is high in fresh fruits and vegetables has been shown to be effective in reducing the risks of a wide array of different types of cancers. As has been noted previously, the Mediterranean diet includes the generous consumption of fresh fruits and vegetables.

The Mediterranean diet includes very little animal fat. There is a direct link between the consumption of animal fat and colorectal cancer, one of the deadliest forms of the disease that oftentimes takes the lives of people in their forties and fifties.

Olive oil (truly the foundation of the Mediterranean diet) had been shown to reduce the risk of breast cancer.

By reducing the risks poised by cancer, the lifespan of men and women has been shown to increase appreciably in studies that have followed groups of people over time.

3. Reducing Coronary Heart Disease Risks

Coronary heart disease is one of the top three causes of premature death throughout the world -- except in the Mediterranean region. Researchers have concluded that diet has played a large and important role in reducing the risk of coronary heart disease amongst the people who populate the countries surrounding the Mediterranean Sea.

An important study in seven countries (Italy, Greece, Yugoslavia, Finland, United States, Netherlands and Japan) demonstrated that those people who followed a Mediterranean diet regimen were less likely to have coronary heart disease and were less likely to have their lives cut short because of serious and ultimately fatal heart conditions.

4. Reducing Hypertension

On some level, the jury is still out on the direct effects between diet and hypertension or high blood pressure. With that said, it clearly has been demonstrated that hypertension and high blood pressure is responsible for premature deaths the world over. In addition, there is strong evidence to suggest that eliminating certain items from a diet -- like processed salts -- can work to reduce the risk of hypertension.

Additionally, there is evidence to support the proposition that a diet high in fiber and low in animal fats (like that of the Mediterranean region) works to reduce the threat of hypertension and premature death from this disease.

5. Diabetes Prevention and Control

The Mediterranean diet is well suited to staving off the serious effects of diabetes. The incidence of premature death because of diabetes is lower in those regions in which the Mediterranean diet is practiced. Because diabetes is a disease that can be controlled through diet, electing to utilize the Mediterranean regimen can work to add literally years to a person's life.

6. The Cumulative Effect of the Mediterranean Diet

It is important to note that the beneficial effects of the Mediterranean diet appear to be cumulative over time. In the other words, the longer a person practices the dining habits of the Mediterranean plan, more of inherent physical benefits of this healthy eating regimen will be ingrained into a person's makeup. Simply put, the benefits of a Mediterranean diet literally are stored up over time, increasing a person's lifespan and adding to his or her overall health and wellbeing not only now, but well into the future.

Mediterranean Diet-Ways to Living a Longer,Without Heart Disease

1. Watch what type of fuel you feed your body

Why do many people buy Super gasoline even though it's more expensive? If they bought the least expensive gas they could save a lot of money. Well, only in the short run. Car engines run more efficiently with high-quality fuels and the parts deteriorate much faster when you use cheap fluids.

Like your car, your body is comprised of different parts and your heart is the engine. The fuel you use to keep your heart and other body parts running makes a difference in your performance, whether you're at work, at school, with your family or anywhere else. It will also affect the speed at which your parts deteriorate.

Nowadays, nutrition experts all over the world are making an effort to introduce the principles of the Mediterranean diet because centuries of experience have proved that it is the best "fuel" available to keep our "parts" running well until old age. Even the European community is recommending this healthy diet to all its members.

2. Cut down on processed foods and load up with fruits and vegetables

To have a healthy heart like the Mediterraneans and maintain normal blood pressure, your diet should be five times higher in potassium than in sodium -the part of salt that is bad for us. Unfortunately, in the typical American diet, the amount of sodium is five times higher than potassium. Why do we have it so backwards? Because seventy-five percent of the salt we eat every day comes from processed foods, most of which is added by manufacturers and restaurants.

Because the American public consumes about 4,000mg per day of sodium, far more than what is needed, the American Public Health Association recently called for a 50 percent sodium reduction in our nation's food supply over the next ten years. It's estimated that such a reduction would save at least 150,000 lives annually.

Fruits and vegetables are low in sodium and high in potassium. By eating fruits and vegetables, you are also replacing other foods in your meals that may be high in sodium. Plus fruits and vegetables contribute good amounts of calcium and magnesium, two minerals that you need for a normal heartrate and to maintain low blood pressure.

3. Give yourself a daily dose of olive oil

Replace saturated fat with extra virgin olive oil. Butter is rarely consumed in the traditional Mediterranean diet and margarine was completely unknown in the area until recently. People in the Mediterranean countries use extra virgin olive oil, one of the best sources of monounsaturated fat, the kind of fat that does not stick to your arteries. Extra virgin olive oil is also an excellent source of many antioxidants such as vitamin E.

If you are considering taking vitamin E in capsules, be aware that you won't get the same results as ingesting extra virgin olive oil. Researchers for the Heart Outcomes Prevention Evaluation Study found that people who received 265 milligrams of vitamin E daily in the form of supplements did not have fewer hospitalizations for heart failure or chest pain when compared to those who received a placebo, a faked pill. That's why nutrition authorities recommend 2 to 3 tablespoons of extra virgin olive oil a day as prevention. So use olive oil and avoid other fat sources such as butter and margarine.

4. Eat more legumes

By legumes, I mean dry beans, lentils, chickpeas and garbanzo beans. Legumes have been a staple food in the Mediterranean diet for centuries. They are packed with minerals such as iron, magnesium, manganese, phosphorous, zinc, potassium, folic acid and some of the B-complex vitamins. They are low in fat and sodium. Legumes are also very high in soluble fiber, which takes cholesterol out of your body through the feces. And to top it all, legumes can help balance your budget because they are very inexpensive. If legumes are not part of your regular diet, you are missing an almost perfect food.

5. Eat more aromatic herbs, garlic and onions

To add the Mediterranean flavor to your meals, replace salt with garlic and aromatic herbs. Garlic is a truly wonder of nature; it has been used for thousands of years as both food and medicine. People around the world, especially those who enjoy fewer chronic heart diseases, use it extensively in their daily diets. Why? Because more than 200 chemical compounds that might protect our bodies have been found in garlic.

Recent studies have shown that garlic can significantly reduce cholesterol and triglycerides, lower blood pressure and prevent the formation of blood clots. It can also protect our bodies through its antioxidant properties.

Onions and other aromatic herbs work very similar to garlic. They contain about 25 active compounds that appear to help combat heart disease, strokes, high blood pressure and cholesterol.

Chapter Seven

Mediterranean Diet Planners

The Mediterranean diet comprises of foods such as cereals, grains, vegetables, dried beans, olive oil, garlic, fresh herbs, seafood, and fruits. Mediterranean diet planners are the nutritionists or dieticians who recommend people with health problems follow a Mediterranean diet.

They plan a specific diet for people with faulty eating habits that can culminate in obesity and other ailments. They focus upon a diet rich in fiber. This intake is naturally contained in fresh herbs, seafood, and fruits and vegetables. People are encouraged to follow a modified Mediterranean diet in which unsaturated fats are substituted with monounsaturated fats, as there is evidence that these ensure longer life expectancy.

Mediterranean diet planners highlight the importance of using olive oil as a cooking medium and dressings for salads. They plan meals that include moderate amounts of fish and meat and low to moderate amounts of cheese and yogurt. They focus on a meal rich in the consumption of fruits, vegetables, potatoes, beans, nuts, seeds, bread and other cereals. The meals also include consumption of wine in moderation.

The diet planners gain information from their patients, before formulating a Mediterranean diet plan for an individual. They acknowledge personal tastes and preferences when they plan a diet for a week or a month. They also make changes in the daily menu, which ensures that the patients are not deprived of their favorite foods and enjoy their daily Mediterranean cuisine with relish.

The planners do not advice people to strictly adhere to the Mediterranean diet but to enjoy a change that rejuvenates their health.

CHOOSE THE RIGHT DIET PLAN - MEDITERRANEAN DIET REVIEW

Choosing Heart-Healthy Options with the Mediterranean Diet

There are many diets out there you can choose from, but for many the Mediterranean diet will be one of the best choices. This is a very healthy diet that can help those with heart issues, high cholesterol, or other health problems. It is an eating plan that will help you discover how to create great tasting meals that are also very good for your heart.

This may be the only diet that includes drinking a glass of red wine, but that has been proven to be very good for your heart. The Mediterranean diet is based around the typical cooking styles of the countries on the coast of the Mediterranean Sea. They love to use olive oil in their cooking, so you can expect to get plenty of good meals made with the health benefits of olive oil.

When you are trying to diet because of the risk of heart disease, it is not as good to use a traditional diet. Even though the same parts, like eating plenty of fruits and vegetables, fish, and whole grains are the same, the Mediterranean Diet helps you take it one step further by giving you the right proportions of the right foods for your heart.

Many studies have been done and they have proven that the traditional Mediterranean Diet will help to reduce the risk of heart disease. This type of diet has also been linked to reduction in cancer, and a reduction in the incidence of Parkinson's and Alzheimer's disease. It is all about good foods cooked in the right ways to keep your heart healthy.

What Does the Mediterranean Diet Emphasize?

There are many things included within the Mediterranean Diet and you need to be aware of what you are getting into. The key components, just like any other diet, are proper eating habits and exercise. In fact, the Mediterranean Diet puts a strong emphasis on getting plenty of exercise each week because this makes a huge difference in heart health.

The Mediterranean Diet also includes eating mainly plant-based foods like vegetables, fruits, legumes, nuts, and whole grains. This does not mean you are a vegetarian on this diet, but you will not be eating as much meat as you may be used to. This diet only calls for eating red meat a few times a month and fish and poultry at least twice a week.

You will also be replacing butter with healthy fats like canola oil and olive oil with this diet. This will help to give your body the fat it needs, but only in the right forms instead of in the bad fats like butter contains. Another big part of the Mediterranean Diet is using herbs and spices instead of salt to flavor your foods.

There is one last component to the Mediterranean Diet and it is the best one of all. It is, of course, optional, but a very large part of the culture of this area of the world and one that many people love. You are supposed to drink red wine in moderation when on the Mediterranean Diet because it is proven a glass of wine with dinner is good for your heart and your body.

Another important part of the diet is enjoying meals with your family and your friends. This is a tradition in the Mediterranean culture and it goes along with the diet. Every component is added because it gives the body the necessary nutrients and it is also very healthy for the heart. This is one of the best diets for anybody with a history of heart disease or high cholesterol.

What I Think About the Mediterranean Diet

Whether you are looking for a healthier way to live and eat or you are looking for a diet to help you lose weight, the Mediterranean Diet is a good choice. You are not going to drop 20 pounds in a month with this diet, but it will help you get to a very healthy weight and maintain it. This is not just a diet you start and finish, but also a way of changing the way you eat every single day for the rest of your life.

It is nice to find a diet that does not completely cut out the things you may enjoy. You can still have red meat, just not that often and you are even encouraged to drink wine with this diet. Most diets do not allow any alcohol and will cut out many of the things you really need. With the Mediterranean Diet, you can have confidence in knowing that you are eating in a hearth healthy way that supports the body completely.

Chapter Eight

Mediterranean Diet Recipes

1. FETA GARBANZO BEAN SALAD

INGREDIENTS

- 1 can (15 ounces) garbanzo beans, rinsed and drained
- 1-1/2 cups coarsely chopped English cucumber (about 1/2 medium)
- 1 can (2-1/4 ounces) sliced ripe olives, drained

- 1 medium tomato, seeded and chopped
- 1/4 cup thinly sliced red onion
- 1/4 cup chopped fresh parsley
- 3 tablespoons olive oil
- 1 tablespoon lemon juice
- 1/4 teaspoon salt
- 1/8 teaspoon pepper
- 5 cups torn mixed salad greens
- 1/2 cup crumbled feta cheese

Total Time

- Prep/Total Time: 15 min.
- Makes
- 4 servings

Directions

Place the first 11 ingredients in a large bowl; toss to combine. Sprinkle with cheese.

Nutrition Facts

2 cups: 268 calories, 16g fat (3g saturated fat), 8mg cholesterol, 586mg sodium, 24g carbohydrate (4g sugars, 7g fiber), 9g protein.

2. COD AND ASPARAGUS BAKE

Ingredients

- 4 cod fillets (4 ounces each)
- 1 pound fresh thin asparagus, trimmed
- 1 pint cherry tomatoes, halved
- 2 tablespoons lemon juice
- 1-1/2 teaspoons grated lemon zest
- 1/4 cup grated Romano cheese

Total Time

- Prep/Total Time: 30 min.
- Makes
- 4 servings

Directions

Preheat oven to 375°. Place cod and asparagus in a 15x10x1-in. baking pan brushed with oil. Add tomatoes, cut side down. Brush fish with lemon juice; sprinkle with lemon zest. Sprinkle fish and vegetables with Romano cheese. Bake until fish just begins to flake easily with a fork, about 12 minutes.

Remove pan from oven; preheat broiler. Broil cod mixture 3-4 in. from heat until vegetables are lightly browned, 2-3 minutes.

Nutrition Facts

1 serving: 141 calories, 3g fat (2g saturated fat), 45mg cholesterol, 184mg sodium, 6g carbohydrate (3g sugars, 2g fiber), 23g protein.

3. SALMON WITH SPINACH & WHITE BEANS

Ingredients

- 4 salmon fillets (4 ounces each)
- 2 teaspoons plus 1 tablespoon olive oil, divided
- 1 teaspoon seafood seasoning
- 1 garlic clove, minced

- 1 can (15 ounces) cannellini beans, rinsed and drained
- 1/4 teaspoon salt
- 1/4 teaspoon pepper
- 1 package (8 ounces) fresh spinach
- Lemon wedges

Total Time

- Prep/Total Time: 15 min.
- Makes
- 4 servings

Directions

Preheat broiler. Rub fillets with 2 teaspoons oil; sprinkle with seafood seasoning. Place on a greased rack of a broiler pan. Broil 5-6 in. from heat 6-8 minutes or until fish just begins to flake easily with a fork.

Meanwhile, in a large skillet, heat remaining oil over medium heat. Add garlic; cook 15-30 seconds or until fragrant. Add beans, salt and pepper, stirring to coat beans with garlic oil. Stir in spinach until wilted. Serve salmon with spinach mixture and lemon wedges.

Nutrition Facts

1 fillet with 1/2 cup spinach mixture : 317 calories, 17g fat (3g saturated fat), 57mg cholesterol, 577mg sodium, 16g carbohydrate (0 sugars, 5g fiber), 24g protein.

4. SKILLET CHICKEN WITH OLIVES

Ingredients

- 4 boneless skinless chicken thighs (about 1 pound)
- 1 teaspoon dried rosemary, crushed
- 1/2 teaspoon pepper
- 1/4 teaspoon salt
- 1 tablespoon olive oil
- 1/2 cup pimiento-stuffed olives, coarsely chopped
- 1/4 cup white wine or chicken broth
- 1 tablespoon drained capers, optional

Total Time

- Prep/Total Time: 20 min.
- Makes
- 4 servings

Directions

Sprinkle chicken with rosemary, pepper and salt. In a large skillet, heat oil over medium-high heat. Brown chicken on both sides.

Add olives, wine and, if desired, capers. Reduce heat; simmer, covered, 2-3 minutes or until a thermometer inserted in chicken reads 170°.

Nutrition Facts

1 serving (calculated without capers): 237 calories, 15g fat (3g saturated fat), 76mg cholesterol, 571mg sodium, 2g carbohydrate (0 sugars, 0 fiber), 21g protein.

5. MEDITERRANEAN PORK AND ORZO

Ingredients

- 1-1/2 pounds pork tenderloin
- 1 teaspoon coarsely ground pepper
- 2 tablespoons olive oil
- 3 quarts water
- 1-1/4 cups uncooked orzo pasta
- 1/4 teaspoon salt
- 1 package (6 ounces) fresh baby spinach
- 1 cup grape tomatoes, halved
- 3/4 cup crumbled feta cheese

Total Time

- Prep/Total Time: 30 min.
- Makes
- 6 servings

Directions

Rub pork with pepper; cut into 1-in. cubes. In a large nonstick skillet, heat oil over medium heat. Add pork; cook and stir 8-10 minutes or until no longer pink.

Meanwhile, in a Dutch oven, bring water to a boil. Stir in orzo and salt; cook, uncovered, 8 minutes. Stir in spinach; cook 45-60 seconds longer or until orzo is tender and spinach is wilted. Drain.

Add tomatoes to pork; heat through. Stir in orzo mixture and cheese.

Nutrition Facts

1-1/3 cups: 372 calories, 11g fat (4g saturated fat), 71mg cholesterol, 306mg sodium, 34g carbohydrate (2g sugars, 3g fiber), 31g protein.

6. GRILLED SQUID

Ingredients

- 800 gr squid

- 2 lemon

- pepper q.s.

- 2 clove garlic

- extra virgin olive oil 1dl

- 50 gr parsley

- Salt to taste

Total Time

- Prep/Total Time: 15 min.

- Makes

- 4 servings

Directions

1) Clean the squid by separating the heads from the body, wash and dry them.

2) Season with salt and a drizzle of oil, cook them on a very hot grill turning them on one side and on the other.

3) Emulsify salt, pepper, parsley and garlic finely chopped with a small glass of oil.

4) Place the squid in a hot dish, season with the sauce and serve with the lemons cut into quarters.

Nutrition facts

Per 100g : 171 calories, 12gr Fat, 3gr carbohydrates, 13gr protein, 71gr water

7. SPAGHETTI OIL, GARLIC AND CHILLI

Ingredients:

- 320gr spaghetti
- garlic 3 cloves

- oil 70gr
- chili pepper 3

Total time

- Prep/Total Time 15 min.
- Makes
- 4 servings

Directions

To prepare spaghetti, garlic, oil and chilli, start by cooking the pasta in boiling salted water to taste.

Cook the spaghetti al dente and in the meantime you can prepare the sauce: peel the garlic cloves, cut them in half and remove the soul (the central green part of each clove).

Reduce the slices into rather thin slices. Take the fresh chilli, and cut it into slices eliminating the stalk. If you prefer a smaller spiciness, you can open it for the sense of length and remove the seeds before reducing it to slices. Now pour the oil into a large pan.

Heat it over a low heat and add the garlic and chilli. Fry the sauce on a very low flame, chilli and garlic will not burn but just fry for a couple of minutes and for a uniform browning without the risk of burning them, you can tilt the pan to collect oil and seasoning in a single point and allow uniform browning. Once the pasta is cooked al dente, you can transfer it directly to the pan and add a ladle of cooking water.

Stir a few moments to mix the flavors and sauté everything, then you can serve your spaghetti with garlic oil and chilli to serve it hot!

Nutrition facts:

for 80gr: Calories 388 kcal, Protein 8.8 g, Carbohydrates 66.4 g, Fat 11.5 g

Conclusions

During the past twenty years, a significant number of people in different countries around the world have turned their attention towards finding healthy diet regimens that are low in saturated fat and that include bountiful servings of fresh fruits and vegetable.

Consequently, the Mediterranean diet has caught the eye of innumerable people who want to include healthy eating into their overall course of prudent living. In short, the Mediterranean diet encompasses foods and beverages that, when consumed in moderation, can work to lessen the threat of some serious diseases and can aid in creating the necessary foundation for a long, hearty lifetime.

The Mediterranean diet is not just a way to lose weight, but is a way to entirely change your life, and in doing so, helping to prolong it. The health benefits are endless, especially when they are combined with exercise, making this nutrition adventure something definitely worth looking into.